Introduction:

Are you tired of dealing with hair loss?

Have you ever thought about giving up on ever having a full head of hair again?

Are you tired of trying to camouflage your thinning hair with haircuts and styles to cover your thinning hairline?

Are you nervous about going outside and getting caught in the rain or worried about that big gust of wind that may expose your hair thinning coverup?

If you are tired of looking in the mirror and not seeing the person you remembered only a few years ago, this book is for you.

I'm going to take you through my personal journey and answer any questions you may have about getting a hair transplant and getting the best results.

I'm going to have some gifts for you in this book that will save you time and money when you are making your decision regarding a hair transplant procedure.

Many of us believe that a small hair transplant with minimal hair grafts should cost a minimum of USD 6000.00 to USD 10,000.00. If you need a large number of hair grafts transplanted, you could expect to pay in upwards of USD 20,000.00 to USD 30,000.00.

This book was written with the information you will need to have up to 5000 hair grafts done for as little as USD 1700.00. Thousands of people globally are accomplishing this now.

TABLE OF CONTENTS

Chapter One

My Hair Loss Journey

Years ago, I decided not to ever shave my head.

I knew I was going to have a challenge with losing my hair as I grew older. My dad had a receding hairline, and on my mother's side, my grandfather and uncle also had a receding hairline. However, I decided not to say "screw it" and shave it all off, as I got older. I knew deep down that someday, with the advancements in hair loss technology, someone would come up with either a cure for hair loss or a cost-effective way to have hair transplanted.

I remember the day I first had someone bring to my attention that my hair was starting to thin. I was sitting in the barber chair, 24 years old, getting my haircut. My hairdresser commented that she was seeing thinning in my hair in the front corners of my head. She asked me what kind of shampoo I was using to wash my hair. I told her I was using "whatever was on sale at the local supermarket." She recommended I use a good quality shampoo and conditioner specially designed for thinning hair to help slow down my hair loss. She said Nioxin, the brand of shampoo and conditioner you will hear me talk about in the next few chapters, makes a product specially designed to help you keep the hair you have. I thought "great" this lady is just trying to sell me her expensive hair products, but what did I have to lose? What I was using wasn't helping my hair loss problem. So that day, I reluctantly bought a bottle of her Nioxin shampoo and conditioner.

The first time I used it, I could tell it was different than the cheap stuff I was using up to then. The instructions on the back of the conditioner said to leave it on the scalp for three minutes before rinsing. After rinsing, my scalp would tingle for several minutes, after drying my hair, I could tell my hair not only felt thicker but looked thicker as well. I've been using Nioxin brand shampoo and conditioner ever since.

At the time of writing this book, I've been using Nioxin #2 for almost twenty years, and I do believe it helps. If you want your hair to be stronger and feel thicker, Nioxin is an excellent product. I would highly recommend giving it a shot. Really when you think about it, using a good quality shampoo and conditioner makes sense. Here's why - today, the conventional theory is that we lose our hair because of testosterone called DHT. DHT is a hormone that squeezes the hair follicles, causing the hair to become thinner and thinner in diameter until the hair stops growing. Nioxin products help your hair stay healthy and thicker, so the hormone DHT has a harder time squeezing the hair follicles resulting in a slowing of the hair loss problem.

If you want to give Nioxin a try for yourself here is a quick rundown of their product:
Nioxin makes a few different types of products.
They categorize their products using a number system. The one I get has Nioxin #2 on the label. Both the shampoo and conditioner towards the bottom of the bottle says, "natural hair progressed hair thinning."

Nioxin shampoo is a cleanser shampoo; it's designed to clean the hair follicles and remove environmental residues on the hair and scalp to keep the hair follicles from clogging. Nioxin conditioner is a scalp therapy conditioner; it is designed to give hair follicles more density, resilience, and controls the moisture balance of your hair and scalp.

Chapter Two

My First Hair Transplant

As time went on, I found myself having to cut my hair shorter and shorter to conceal my hair thinning. It seemed like the shorter the sides of my hair were, the less thin the top of my hair seemed to look. By now, I was starting to buy and wear more hats. Hats seemed like the best way to cover my thinning hair. If you are losing your hair, you know what I mean, it just feels like there is a piece of you is missing. It's like in your mind you see yourself one way, but when you look in the mirror, it turns into a big let down. It's like you know that it's coming because your dad and grandfather are balding, but you're just hoping and praying it's going to skip you. The worst thing about it is it seems to change you emotionally as a person; you don't seem quite as happy and lose some self-confidence. Everything about it sucks!

I remember one day a friend of mine asked me if I wanted to get some discounts on ski tickets from the local college. He said all we have to do is go in, and they'll give us a particular ID that would allow us to get discounts through the college. I said, "Wow, that sounds great; let's do it." That week, as my wife was sitting dinner on the table, a big juicy ribeye steak with a big salad, my buddy called and said, "Tomorrow, let's go and get those IDs from the college." I said, "Yeah okay," not really paying attention, since I was focusing on sinking my teeth into that ribeye steak. The next morning, I was running late for work and forgot we were supposed to meet that afternoon. So instead of taking the time to fix my hair, I threw on a hat and ran out the door. That afternoon my buddy came by the office and said, "let's head over there real quick and get those IDs made up." I said "okay" while in the back of my mind thinking - it shouldn't be a big deal to wear a hat for my picture.

We arrived at the college. As we're walking up to the desk, we were greeted by two young college girls. My buddy says he was there to get some ID's made up so that we can get discounts on lift tickets. I think my buddy knew the girls because they were all smiles.

To this day, I still don't know if they were doing him a favor or not. Anyhow the girl said, "follow me"; they took us over to a room that had a white screen backdrop with a small chair sitting in front of it. My buddy went up, took a quick picture, and then followed one of the girls out to get his ID. Now it was my turn. I sat down on the stool, and the first thing the girl says is "please take your hat off." I was thinking to myself "oh great! Who knows what this mess is going to look like." I took my hat off quickly, feeling a big pit in my stomach thinking to myself I probably looked 25 with my hat on, but with it off - it was like I was 45. I can still remember the young college student handing me the ID card with a picture of me, my hair matted down, and the receding hair at my temples.

This episode was a big turning point for me. Over the following week, I started looking up hair transplant companies around the USA on the Internet. One of the ones that kept showing up was Bosley Hair Restoration & Transplant. They seemed to have the most experience. I called them up and asked, "What do you guys typically charge for a hair transplant?" They were charging approximately USD 9.50 per hair graft but did not know how many graphs I would need without an in-person consultation. I could choose an appointment for a consultation at either their office in Phoenix, Arizona, or Denver, Colorado.

That day I scheduled to have the examination done the following week in Denver, Colorado, at the Bosley Office. The next week I made the trip to Denver. The address they gave me was to an office at a high-rise in downtown Denver.

Going up the elevator, I thought, "well, at least they're located in Denver, so I don't have to travel too far to have the hair transplant procedure done." In my mind, I pictured a big office with a secretary and a waiting room like most medical clinics. I thought it would be kind of like a dentist's office or something similar. After reaching the floor, I exited in the elevator and noticed there was just a long hallway with a bunch of small doors. I walked down the hall, passing several doors and finally got to the one that said Bosley Hair Restoration & Transplant on it.

I walked in and was greeted by a middle-aged man; he said: "I'll be the one doing your consultation." Over the next 30 minutes or so, he took a look at what he called my "donor area," he explained to me how the procedure is done. He explained the doctor would cut a strip of skin that contained hair follicles from the back of my head. The doctor and his assistants would dissect each hair follicle to be transplanted back into the thin or balding areas of my head. With small incisions in the front of my head, they would transplant each hair follicle. He recommended that I do a minimum of 800 hair grafts. He also said that they would do a minimal reconstruction of my hairline, but would focus more on adding density to the areas that were thinning.

I said, "Ok, so how much is this going to cost me? And how long does the procedure take?" He says, "Well, I have good news and bad news... the good news is we're running a special we're only charging USD 9.00 per hair graft, the bad news is that the procedure cannot be done at the Denver office. We have two offices on the west coast that you can choose from - one is in Los Angeles, California, and the other one is in Scottsdale, Arizona."

I think to myself - I don't have this kind of money to spend on my hair. Then he proceeds to say, "we have financing options available." I said, "give me whatever information you have for me, and I will have to talk over with my wife."

So at this point to do 800 hair grafts it's USD 7200.00 and to do 1000 hair grafts, it's USD 9000.00.
Plus, I have to add the extra expenses of travel, hotel, food, and extras to travel from Colorado USA to Arizona USA for the hair transplant procedure.

Then I started dreaming about how awesome it would be to have all of my hair back. All I could think about on the way home was how am I going to convince my wife that it would be worth spending the USD 7000.00-9000.00 on an 800 to 1000 hair transplant.
When I get home, my wife looks at me with a small smirk on her face and says, "Well, how much is it?" After a good solid hour of

discussing all the details. I come up with a brilliant idea.

At the time we owned a Full-Service Glass Shop in Southern Colorado. We started the business from scratch.

Our company was about four years old, and we were growing. When we first started the business, we decided that I would get a small personal allowance of USD 200.00 per month over and above our wages with the company. I was free to spend my allowance on anything I wanted. All other monies went right back into our growing business.

So by now, you can probably tell what my brilliant idea was. My suggestion was to go for the finance option, and put all of my monthly allowance into paying the hair transplant loan as quickly as possible."

Personally, having my hair back was worth sacrificing three years of personal spending allowance. So the following week, we scheduled to have the procedure done at their Scottsdale, Arizona location.

Chapter Three

The Procedure

The big day had finally arrived. I was a bit nervous. Just the thought of having a strip of skin being cut and removed from the back of my head seemed a little bit unnerving. But because I had seen many guys that had already had the procedure done, my confidence was restored. They had provided testimonials with before and after pictures, which showed excellent results. After seeing all the social proof, I realized I was probably just overthinking this. Surely I had nothing to worry about.

For the procedure, we traveled to Scottsdale, Arizona to a high-end area located northeast of Phoenix. The procedure was to take place inside another office building. However, this time, it was almost exactly what I pictured. It was like a dentist's office, but bigger. When I first got there, I met with a doctor and what appeared to be a consultant or salesperson for Bosley. They once again went over all the details with me of what exactly the procedure entailed.

Here's a quick breakdown of the procedure. They were going to inject the back and the top of my head with some local anesthesia to numb the entire area. Then the doctor would remove 3/8 "to 1/2" strip of skin containing all the hair follicles. Next to the doctor would sew up the incision, and his assistant would begin immediately to dissect each hair follicle from the strip. The doctor would then give his assistant some time to cut each hair follicle carefully. Then the doctor would come back in, make small cuts in my scalp, and his assistant would place each hair follicle into the tiny cuts in my scalp.

Being that we decided to go with the finance option, we originally qualified for 800 hair grafts, the minimum they recommended. Like I said, though, they had me meet with a consultant or salesperson and the doctor initially. The salesperson notified me I was approved to finance 800 hair grafts. However, since I made the trip from Colorado to Arizona, they highly recommended that I get at least 1000 hair grafts.   Reasoning that throughout time I would lose more hair and possibly need a second hair transplant.

After doing the math quickly, I realized that another 200 hair grafts would cost about USD 1800.00, so I agreed, and we moved forward on the procedure. I hopped on the phone with the loan company and was approved for another 200 hair grafts that would make a total of 1000 hair grafts for my first hair transplant.

All in all, it was a pretty good experience. The needles that they use to administer the anesthesia were quite painful; however, when the anesthesia started kicking in, I didn't feel anything, but pressure for the rest of the procedure. The procedure took a good day, around 6 hours. They even ordered me lunch from a local restaurant.

Once everything was complete, I had a white bandage wrapped around my head to protect the stitches on the back of my scalp. Then they sent me on my way with some shampoo they recommend, along with some oral pills of Propecia, painkillers, and some antibiotics.

After the initial anesthesia wore off, I remember some pain, especially around the area that they took the strip at the back of my head. I also had some bruising, and my eyes got black for a couple of days. I did take some painkillers, and that helped with the pain. I came back the following day for them to remove the bandages and do a thorough examination of the stitches, making sure there was no infection. The part that I did not like was the back of my head remained numb, and it stayed that way for several months.

In most cases, when you have a hair transplant, the hair in the transplanted follicle will fall out, then right behind it, a new hair will start to grow. That is what they call shedding. I only had a few hair follicles that actually fell out; it seemed like the rest of them just grew and didn't shed.

I tried their shampoo for a few days, but I didn't like it. It seemed to make my scalp itchy, so I went back to using Nioxin #2 shampoo and conditioner. I'm convinced that was a way better option than using the shampoo they gave me. Also, Propecia pills they gave me I tried a few, but I had some weird side effects, so I did not keep taking them.

Within four to five months, I had new hair with some length to it growing in, and all my bald spots started to fill-in. It's incredible when you get your hair back.   I think the best part of it is - it's one less thing that's taking up space in your brain. You stop thinking about it. There's just something about it that changes you! Adds more confidence to your step.

Chapter Four

Thirteen years later

I was 30 years old when I got my first hair transplant and was pretty confident that my hair was going to continue to reseed over the years. Knowing this I've continued to use the Nioxin #2 shampoo and conditioner. I do believe that helps slow the hair loss. My hair loss is almost identical to my father's hair loss. His hair loss is receded about halfway back on his head, and the front is smooth. But with my hair loss, I've been able to maintain a small percentage of my hair to about halfway back on my head. So it appears that after 13 years, I still have close to the 1000 transplanted hairs that I originally had done during the Bosley procedure.

I want to go through the different phases I went through over the last 13 years following my first hair transplant procedure. My first hair transplant took about five to six months for my hair to start coming back in. Then over the next five years, everything seemed to stay pretty consistent between the density and thickness of my transplanted hair.

After those first five, though, it seemed like every year, I would lose just a little bit more density. In 2015 it was getting to the point where I was contemplating getting a second hair transplant. I started researching to see if there was any new technology out there since the last time I researched.

The first thing I found was a doctor in Florida USA area who was known for extracting individual follicles instead of cutting a strip out from the back of your head. The exciting thing about this was once the procedure is complete, it would be hard to tell that you had follicles removed. The beautiful thing about having it done that way would be that you could shave the back your head without any signs of having a hair transplant. The problem was that it was still going to be a costly procedure. I also wanted to get a lot more than just 1000 hair grafts.

So I kept digging. I found a relatively new technology that I've heard about before, but it is not being used for hair growth. This method is fascinating to me; it's like a maintenance procedure called PRP treatment.

PRP is an exciting advancement in the medical industry; it stands for platelet-rich plasma. It's a process where a small amount of blood is drawn from your vein. The blood is collected in blood collection tubes and then transfer it into a centrifuge machine that spins it and separates the platelet-rich plasma from the rest of the blood. The Platelet Rich Plasma, also known as PRP is then injected into your scalp.

The PRP is the stuff your body uses when healing a cut, so it provides nutrients and increases the blood vessels in the area where the PRP is injected. This process revitalizes the scalp, enabling hairs that are being squeezed out from the THC hormone to start growing again. This technology is excellent; however, it is quite expensive and has to be administered at least once or twice a year to maintain results.

So at this point, I'm still thinking of just doing another hair transplant instead. Something else that kept coming up in my research for solutions to thinning hair was a weird product that appeared to be colored dust that guys were sprinkling in their hair to make their hair appear thicker. I thought that's the most ridiculous thing I've ever seen. It did not make sense. However, I started seeing pictures of guys before and after, and the results looked pretty good.

So I went to Amazon to see what it cost. It was quite expensive, being a powder at USD 59.00 per ounce. They had a sample bottle that was only a few dollars, so I thought "I'll buy it for kicks and see if it proves my assumptions wrong."

A few days later, it came in the mail, and that evening after getting out of the shower, I thought I'll give it a shot. I sprinkled a bit of it on the area of my head where the hair was thinning, patted the area lightly with my hand, and the thinning area seemed to disappear. The color was soft black, and it matched perfectly.

Still in the back of my mind, there is no way this is working as good as I thought it was. I call for my wife, Rachel, to come and check it out. At first, she looked and told me to turn around, and then she wanted to see the top. I said, "okay, what do you think?" She looked at me, her eyebrows raised and she said: "looks good - it doesn't look like you put anything in it." I was blown away by the results.

At this point, I thought I'm going to get another hair transplant soon, so I'll use this stuff until I get my next hair transplant. It sounded like a good plan. Then I started thinking of everything that could go wrong. What if a big gust of wind came up and blew this stuff out of my hair? Solution: hairspray, use some good hairspray; it locks everything in place.

In heavy winds, light rain, and even one time in Cancun Mexico, we went on an excursion riding underwater motorbikes, they put the bikes in the water fully immersed. On the bikes was a large round helmet where they pump oxygen into the helmet. So they had us swim to the bike then duck our heads under the water then up into the large helmet. I was thinking, "Great, I'm going to go under the water, and all of this hair stuff is going to wash out." So I went under as quick as I could, I was maybe two seconds immersed when I came into the helmet filled with oxygen, I reached my hand up and wiped my forehead, there was no black residue on my hand, so I thought well maybe it didn't come off.

We finished the excursion taking pictures and everything. Then we had to exit the same way being fully immersed under the water for 1 to 2 seconds. I swam back to the boat, climbed up the ladder, went to the area where I was keeping my stuff, and threw a hat on. I asked Rachel, my wife, if she noticed if all the hair stuff washed out when we were inside the helmet of the motorbike she said she didn't notice and everything worked out fine.

Later on that day, when we got to the hotel, I took my hat off to see how it looked, and it appeared that the hairspray kept everything intact. I think it was because I was using humidity-resistant hairspray, and being fully submerged under the water for only a few seconds didn't affect it at all; it just matted my hair down, which wasn't a big deal. This stuff is fascinating. It wasn't a powder. It's like little tiny particles of micro hairs- this is the only way I can describe it. It comes in a small plastic container, almost like a salt and pepper shaker.

If you would like to see how I use it, I'll put some videos in our Confidential Facebook group. Here is the link to request to be added to the group
www.TheHairTransplantBook.com/Support-Links

Chapter Five

Hair transplants at a fraction of the cost.

I went in for a hair transplant consultation two years ago with a company in Orlando, Florida. The following is what they recommended to get a full head of hair. First, they wanted me to get 1800 hair grafts. Immediately before the hair treatment, they wanted to do a PRP treatment. They said this would ensure that all of the hair grafts would take at 98 to 99% success rate. They were also going to tattoo the scar I had on the back of my head from the previous hair transplant. The tattooing process is relatively new; it's like microdots to replicate hair follicles and camouflage the scar making it appear to have hair growing there. They wanted to do all this for the one low price of USD 12,000.00.

As you read the rest of this chapter, I want you to remember the prices above. Now things get interesting, about six months later, the same place in Orlando, Florida contacted me and said they were running a special. (It must've been their slow season). They said they could do all 1800 hair grafts for half the price of USD 6000.00. I thought wow, this is an awesome price. Half price! There was no way I was going to pass this up. Half price, and I could have a full head of hair back!

Remember my first hair transplant was only 1000 hair grafts, and it didn't include PRP or anything extra. My first hair transplant cost me USD 9000.00 - now 13 years later they're telling me they can do it at 1800 hair graphs and fix my scar and do PRP treatment for only USD 6000.00!!! I mean come on how can I pass this one up. However, I was not able to get away to have it done due to some other family commitments at the time. The other challenge was that we were back in Colorado, and the half-off procedure was offered at the office in Orlando Florida.

My wheels were turning. I started thinking: WOW they were willing to drop this treatment to half price. I wonder if there are other people out there doing the same thing. Maybe a hair transplant is much easier than I imagined if they were willing to take that much of a loss.

There's got to be a lot of profit built into their profit margins for hair transplants.

Several weeks later during a trip, my wife and I started discussing different options. It was at that point I had remembered years ago a colleague of ours was into medical tourism; he had a business built around it. So my wife and I started looking up what the hair transplant procedure cost is in different parts of the world. We started seeing there were places around the world that were known for hair transplants.

One of the locations that kept coming up was in the country of Turkey, especially Istanbul, Turkey. As we researched, we found out that Istanbul, Turkey has over 350 clinics that do hair transplants. Prices range from USD 500.00 up to USD 3000.00 to get 5000 hair grafts done.

Equivalent procedures like this in the United States would range anywhere from USD 10,000 to USD 30,000. We also learned that Istanbul, Turkey has state-of-the-art medical facilities, and many of their doctors are educated and some even coming from other countries around Europe. They are using all the same technology and techniques used throughout Europe and the USA. With this knowledge, my wife and I started contacting various clinics in Turkey; specifically, Istanbul, checking on customer ratings and verified testimonials, that caught our attention.

After receiving numerous quotes and complete medical tourism packages from the clinics in Istanbul, I'll cover what they included in their cost package. Each package ranges anywhere from USD 1700.00 up to USD 2500.00; here's where it gets interesting.

I'm now planning on going to Istanbul, Turkey within the next month to have a hair transplant procedure done. The cost we've been quoted is anywhere from USD 1700.00 to around USD 2500.00. That's a great price, right? However, that price is for a medical package deal, and here's what's included: the hair transplant procedure, transportation from the airport to the hotel, your hotel stay for two to four nights, free breakfast, and all of your transportation back-and-forth from the hotel to the clinic for your appointments. So you're not only getting the hair transplant, but you are getting several hundred dollars in extras for lodging, transportation, and a translation assistant. So actually these hair transplants are costing less than USD 2000.00 in most cases. That, to me, is just mind-blowing.

I now live in Colorado Springs, Colorado, I'm finding flights from Colorado Springs Airport to Istanbul, Turkey (IST Airport Code) round-trip for around USD 750.00.

So I can fly to Istanbul Turkey, stay in a four or five-star hotel, receive a hair transplant with up to 5000 hair grafts with PRP treatment, transportation, a personal international translation assistant who looks after me throughout my stay and still spend less than USD 3500.00.

Now when I started to talk to family and friends about going to Istanbul, several of them were a little freaked out, saying, "Really? I'd be careful if you're going to go there." I guess Turkey in past years, has had some bad publicity. Any time you travel to a foreign country it is vital that you travel smart, especially in the big cities. Istanbul is the largest city in Turkey and even though precautions should be taken, the city has been a safe place for global visitors seeking medical procedures. A large part of their population is in their 20s and 30s and has mellowed over the past several years and is welcoming to medical tourism.

If you would like to see videos for my travels to Turkey, I will be taking lots of videos documenting us exploring the area along with the hair transplant procedure.
You can go here
www.TheHairTransplantBook.com/Support-Links to gain access to our confidential Facebook group.

Different countries around the world charge the following average cost for hair transplants:
(Cost Based on Research 9-2019)
Turkey USD 1,735.00
Hungry USD 2,600.00
India USD 2,800.00
Ireland USD 12,000.00
Malaysia USD 3,640.00
Poland USD 3,900.00
Germany USD 3300.00
Thailand USD 3,350.00
Mexico USD 3,700.00
UAE USD 5,445.00
United Kingdom USD 8,100.00
United States USD 7,900.00

Chapter Six

Harvesting Hair and Best options

Where can hair be transplanted and harvested from the body, and what are the best hair transplant options?

There are a few different types of hair transplants.
First, let's explore where can hair be transplanted from on your body for a hair transplant procedure.

Hair can be taken from various parts of the body and be transplanted to just about anywhere on the body. For instance, some people want to fill in their eyebrows; others may want to fill in their beard area. Most want a hair transplant done for the top front part of the head and or the top back part commonly referred to as the crown of the head. There are three main areas in which hair is most often transplanted from. The first is the very back and side portion of the head, the side of your head that wraps around to the ears - is the main donor area. The second is the front of the neck - this is the hairs from the beard of your face. The third donor area is body hair - this hair is mainly the chest and back area. These are the three most common donor areas used for extracting hair to be transplanted.

In the hair transplant clinics of today, there is a variety of new methods being used to not only extract the hair follicles but new ways to transplant each hair follicle.

When I had mine done 13 years ago, the top clinics were only offering one kind of procedure — commonly known as the strip procedure.

Throughout the surgical hair transplant industry, it is frequently called FUT "follicular unit transplantation," here is a quick recap of a FUT procedure. First, a strip of skin is cut and removed from the back of your head then the gap where the piece is removed is sutured back together. Many physicians will argue that they like the strip method because it allows a larger amount of hair grafts to be extracted in one procedure. They claim it is less expensive and has less of an impact on the patient's donor area.

In October 2019, I had a consultation here in Colorado USA with a widely recognized company that I won't mention. They tried to convince me to go with another strip procedure consisting of a hair transplant of only 1200 hair grafts.

I asked their method of transplanting the hair grafts into the new balding area, they explained they still used the same methods they were using 13 years ago, when I had my first hair transplant done. This method consisted of the doctor making the thousand or so small cuts into the skin using a small steel blade. Then they would have their medical assistant carefully place the hair graphs into each cut or incision. When the physician told me this, I was shocked that they were still using this old, outdated technology. I had done a ton of research and had numerous consultations and proposals from hair restoration clinics all over the world.

The strip procedure/ FUT is still common for people that are experiencing severe balding. However, there are several new ways of transplanting the new hair follicles into the balding area of your body.

The new ways consist of using different types of medical pens to relocate the hair follicle, they load each hair follicle into the pen and then transplant it into the desired area during the procedure. Doing it this new way allows for the clinical technician to place the hair grafts tighter together, especially in the front hairline area, to give the patient a more natural hairline. It also is less trauma to the hair transplant area to use the new medical pen technology. These new styles of hair transplant procedures are, in my opinion, the best way to get your desired results.

I have quite a bit of sales experience under my belt and have conducted a lot of business in the USA market, and I can say that I understand sales at a higher level than most. I can tell when somebody's trying to "sell" me.

With that said, from the last few consultations I've had in the USA, this is my impression. I believe that several of these large corporate companies in the USA are using outdated technology because most people are not educated about what is actually available on a global scale.

This was a significant takeaway I had from my last consultation. After checking my donor area, the sales consultant said she thought I should get around 1800 hair grafts done. However, when the physician came in, she looked at my donor area and recommended only doing 1600 hair grafts. When the salesperson asked her why she reduced the number of hair grafts, she said: "Because the scar from the last procedure is a little bit wide on the ends, and the amount of hair that can be harvested will be less than expected during the second hair transplant."

From an economic standpoint if I could convince you into coming back to me three times and having a strip procedure done only giving you 1000 to 1500 grafts for USD 9000.00 to USD 10,000.00 per time that means

I would make USD 30,000.00 over the years and would have only transplanted 3000 to 4500 hairs. Their BIG profits are made in recommending multiple small procedures. Sometimes this process is necessary as in the case of you just starting to lose your hair showing noticeable effects of a receding hairline. However, if you are at what the industry refers to as a Norwood seven or six or even five having to go back to have three, four or even five different procedures can be quite costly.

When in the process of performing a new strip procedure hair transplant a second time, the new strip they cut would contain the old scar, therefore automatically giving them fewer hair follicles for the second hair transplant.

So think about that for a minute, the scar from the strip procedure automatically reduces the number of hair grafts available for the next hair transplant procedure. I believe this is a big contradiction from the arguments I've heard of mostly USA doctors. The reason they give for not doing the FUE or follicular unit extraction is that it harms the donor area and can potentially leave patchy areas on the scalp at the scar area.

I believe it's because they have little to no experience here in the USA doing FUE procedures. From the research I've done, it appears to take a lot of skill and hand-eye coordination, when performing a traditional FUE. FUE is very labor-intensive.

The clinic I consulted with located in Orlando, Florida was the only clinic in the USA that was doing FUE. However, they were using a robotic arm to do it. Doing it this way automatically takes the labor-intensive part out of the equation, and having trained medical staff who are capable of the techniques and skills necessary to complete a successful FUE hair transplant procedure is paramount.

The only problem I have with the robotic arm when performing FUE hair transplant procedure is the tool they use has to cut the skin area around each hair follicle mechanically. So it would make sense that a robotic arm would be able to make a precise cut, right? However, the hair follicles grow out of the skin a variety of angles, if the robotic arm cut around the hair follicle is not at the right angle it will damage the hair follicle and possibly other hair follicles next to it.

This is one reason I am a firm believer in having a human perform the FUE procedure. I believe it is a better option. My other argument is the FUE procedure is very challenging when performed on people with extremely curly hair because the hair grows at different angles and is very difficult to extract hair grafts effectively. This is the one case that, in my opinion, would require a FUT (strip procedure) is if you have naturally curly hair.

If you're not sure, you could always send your pictures to the clinic to evaluate your hair type and find out what they would recommend. If you do decide to go with the FUT (strip procedure), keep in mind, this procedure will leave you with a small linear scar around the back of your head.

Two ways to hide a lineal scar from FUT (Strip Procedure)

When having a FUT hair transplant procedure, the doctor must be skilled at suturing the skin back together. It is also vital that you do not engage in any strenuous exercises for several weeks. Doing so can stress the skin of the strip area healing around the scar and cause the area to stretch, creating a more prominent scar. Your objective should be to keep the scar tight until it's fully healed, so it will be as unnoticeable as possible.

The way to cover your scar is always to keep your haircut around the scar a length of approximately one-half inch.

I cut my hair like this; however, for some reason, my scar is a little bit wider towards the end of the scar from my first hair transplant. So I have these two small areas approximately 1 inch or so on each side of my head that generally show just a little bit.

The second method works great. If you have a desire to cut your hair shorter than 1/2 inch, there is a procedure referred to in the industry as micro-pigmentation. It's a perfect way of camouflaging the scar from a hair transplant.

It consists basically of micro tattoos that are tattooed to the scar. These micro tattoos replicate the look of small hair follicles, which surprisingly can make the scar virtually disappear. Although this procedure works great, there are a couple of details you need to be aware of when searching for someone to perform it. First, make sure you find someone that can perform this procedure once without having to do it multiple times. There are only specific needles that work great for creating the perfect appearance of a replicated hair follicle. If they are not using the special needles, they would have to perform the procedure multiple times to get the desired results.

One of the consultations I had at a well-known hair restoration clinic here in the USA said they charge an outrageous price of USD 1500.00 just to perform micro-pigmentation on a scar that is only approximately 9 inches long. They said it would take multiple appointments to complete the procedure. This is an immediate red flag not to use them and go elsewhere for the procedure. Make sure to ask to see results from other patients they have performed this procedure on. When done correctly, it should look exactly like small dots replicating the hair follicles that are the exact color of your hair. I've seen some bad jobs out there where the pigment appears washed out and is even a bluish-green color like a lousy tattoo job.

The second type of extraction procedure is known as FUE or -follicular unit extraction. FUE is where either a medical professional using a specialty tool or a machine robot extracts each hair follicle. This is a relatively new method of extracting hair follicles but opens up access to other donor areas from various parts of the body, donor areas not limited to just the head donor area but the neck, chest or back. Being that it is mildly invasive, once the donor area is healed, it is virtually impossible to detect that hair has been taken from the donor area.

Each hair follicle transplanted can contain as little as one and up to four hairs per follicle.

Next, let's go over the options available to transplant hair into the recipient area.

When positioning each hair follicle, there are two different ways they can be transplanted. One is where the doctor makes tiny incisions into the scalp angling them if necessary to meet your hair pattern. Then medical technicians come in and slowly place each follicle into the micro incisions made by the doctor. Using this method makes it more challenging to place the follicles in a tight pattern unless it is done using a sapphire blade. The other method is called DHI. In this method, a tool that is in the shape of a pen is used. The medical technician loads each hair follicle into this pen-like tool. Then another medical technician uses the pen-like tool to insert and angle each hair follicles into the scalp. This method is much more effective at positioning the hair follicles tighter together, resulting in a more natural-looking hairline. There are also many benefits to this that we'll cover later.

Chapter Seven

What stage of hair loss are you at now?

Several factors come into play when it comes to determining how effective a hair transplant will be. The first thing you want to consider is how big the donor area is. The size of the donor area can be determined by how severe your existing hair loss is.

There are many indicators to tell what the final severity of your hair loss will be. Some say it comes from the mother's side of the family. Another hypothesis I've heard that makes the most sense is, if your facial features are that of your fathers, then you will most likely have the same hair growth patterns as him or his side of the family. However, if it doesn't, then you will most likely inherit the hair growth pattern of your mother's side of the family.

The other factor that determines whether you will have a successful hair transplant is the thickness and density of your hair. The thicker your existing hair is, the more likely you are to have a more significant amount of hair follicles with multiple strands of hair per hair follicle. As previously stated, hair follicles grow in groups of 1,2,3 and 4 hairs per follicular hair unit.

Below is a chart that the hair transplant industry calls the Norwood scale. This chart will help you identify which stage of hair loss you were at and or have the potential to be in the future.

This Norwood scale is important because it will help you identify patterns. It will also give you the ability to determine what your final inherited hair pattern will look like if you do nothing to fix it. The Norwood scale will also help you communicate better with the doctors and or clinics when discussing the treatment that is the best option for you. In most cases, it is an excellent idea to let them know where on the Norwood scale, and where you see yourself being in 5, 10, or 20 years from now.

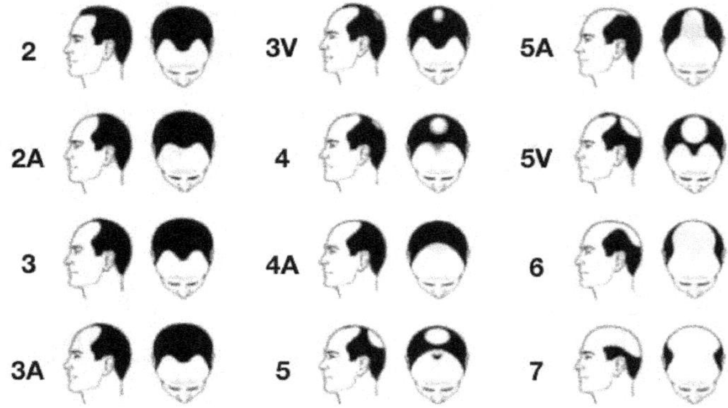

2
2A
3
3A
3V
4
4A
5
5A
5V
6
7

Chapter Eight

Procedure Options Overview

The following are some of the industry's terminology and abbreviations you will want to learn while embarking on this journey of hair transplantation.
FUE, FUT, DHI, BHT, PRP, Mesotherapy, sapphire tool, and artist robotic arm

Let's cover them one by one:

FUE, this stands for follicular unit extraction. You will hear FUE thrown around a lot when people are talking about hair transplant procedures. Many will refer to the whole hair transplant as FUE. Don't let it confuse you. FUE is strictly the method used for extracting each hair follicle. FUE has nothing to do with the method used for placing and distributing each of the extracted follicles back into the area for the hair transplant.

You will also hear terms used like Micro FUE.

Micro FUE is a series of punches that are like small cylindrical shaped blades that are used to extract each hair follicle almost like a cookie-cutter on a micro-scale.

There are also several types of extraction punches. There are punches that spin and punches that don't, There are rotary or non-rotary. The extraction punches that spin has a small motor attached to them that makes them spin. The other type of rotary punches are designed to have the medical technician physically spin the punch instead of a motor. Just imagine having to twist a screwdriver quickly several thousand times. Yeah, I don't want that procedure done on me. I think it would get tiring to physically spin the punch with your hand, especially if you are having thousands of hair graph extractions.
In my opinion, this would make the procedure vulnerable to a high rate of human error. Therefore, I would highly recommend finding a clinic that uses a motorized rotary punch, when performing the FUE procedure.

FUT stands for (follicular unit transplantation).

This is one of the original methods used to remove the hair follicles from the donor area, commonly known as the strip method. It is called the strip method because a small strip of skin is cut and removed from the donor area in the back of your head. The strip of skin is commonly 1cm wide and spans from one side of your head to the other, usually just above and to the back of each ear. This method always leaves a scar, and hopefully not be a big scar as long as you have an excellent doctor stitching it back together.

DHI stands for (Direct Hair Implant)

DHI referred strictly to the method of placing the transplanted hair follicles back into the skin once extracted. This procedure is done with medical tools commonly known as an Implanter Pen or Choi Pen. To date, this method has been determined to be the least invasive way of transplanting the new hair follicles. Using the implanter pen allows the physician or medical technician to transplant the hair follicles in a tighter pattern giving the patient a more natural-looking hairline as a result. There's less trauma to the transplanted area resulting in a faster healing time and less chance of disturbing any of the remaining native hair. This method also allows hair to be transplanted without having to shave the head. Hair follicles can be transplanted in about two or three minutes after the extraction process, reducing the time that they remain outside of the body. The drawback? This procedure is usually a little bit more expensive, simply because it is more labor-intensive. Typically one person will carefully position and insert the hair follicles into the recipient area. At the same time, two or three other medical assistants will carefully load each one of the implanter pens with the hair follicles that were recently extracted from the donor area.

BHT stands for (Body Hair Transplant)
When I first heard of this, I was a bit skeptical. However, many of the clinics we have reached out to in Istanbul, Turkey gave the option of BHT. I have chatted with several people that have had it done and have seen some tremendous personal results. Many results from people getting 6000 to 7000 hair grafts. BHT may be recommended if you are at a

Norwood six or seven and have a weak donor area. Body hair transplants are typically taken from the beard, specifically the area under the chin and the neck. The other commonplace for hair extraction is the chest area.

Sapphire tool

The sapphire tool is one of several different tools used to create small incisions or channels in the skin for the placement of individual hair follicles. In the past, it was common to use steel blades; however, sapphire blades leave a smaller, almost perfectly shaped channel. This channel enables the medical doctor to position each follicle giving a more dense result.

Some clinics will recommend using DHI in front of the hairline, where it is especially important to create a denser thick, natural look. Then recommend using the sapphire blade on the other areas during the hair transplant.

PRP (Platelet Rich Plasma)

PRP is a natural substance the body produces that can be extracted from your own blood. The doctor draws one or two vials of blood from you; he puts it into a machine that quickly spins it. This process separates the blood and makes the PRP rise to the top. This PRP is what your body uses when it is in the process of healing a cut on your skin. PRP naturally increases the blood flow to the area and gives it the necessary building blocks to help the body repair itself. Since PRP increases nutrients to the area where it is injected, it gives your hair the strength required to resist the effects of DHT, the testosterone that strangles the hair follicles.

There are several benefits that come from this. First, if you have thinning hair, the PRP will help thicken it naturally. Second, if you have peach fuzz hair that does not want to seem to grow, PRP will help give it the strength to grow in thicker. If you're at the point that you're getting a hair transplant, it is recommended to go with a clinic that incorporates PRP in the hair transplant process. The clinics that include PRP can guarantee a higher percentage rate of transplanted hair. PRP is reasonably new in the hair transplant industry, however, it's one of the best-kept secrets. Since it's coming from your own body and is not a drug, and there are no side effects.

Mesotherapy

Mesotherapy is a treatment that consists of a series of injections. Traditionally the injections have a unique formula of vitamins, enzymes, hormones, and plant-based extracts. This formula is designed to rejuvenate and tighten the skin. The idea behind Mesotherapy is that it helps correct underlying issues like poor circulation and inflammation that can cause skin damage. Some medical professionals also use Mesotherapy to inject finasteride and minoxidil. The clinic I have recently chosen to do my second hair transplant proposed to use Mesotherapy in combination with PRP - Platelet Rich Plasma, during my next hair transplant procedure.

If you would like to see the video vlogs I have done documenting my complete journey from start to finish, it will be published and available in our Confidential Facebook group. www.TheHairTransplantBook.com/Support-Links

Robotic and Artas Robotic for Hair Transplants

There are a few different modern robotic hair transplant systems that are capable of performing a large part of a single hair transplant procedure. The most common one in the USA is the ATRAS. I first heard about this procedure referred to as a robot assistant. It was about a year ago, in 2018 when I went for a consultation with a company located in Orlando, Florida. I have to admit that when I first heard of the concept, I was extremely excited. I thought, wow, I can not believe how far technology has come over the past 13 years since I had my first procedure. I thought having a robot cherry-pick each hair graft would be a great advancement for hair transplants. I mean, it sounds good. Robot technology claims that the robot zeros in on only hair follicles that contain 2, 3, and 4 hair follicles making it possible to double or triple your hair transplant results.

Robot Drawbacks

ARTAS robotic technology is only licensed to extract hair follicles in dark-haired patients with straight hair. The disadvantage is that men with blonde, red, or grey hair face is that they must first dye their hair to allow the robotic system to work correctly.

However, even dark-haired people can have different shades of hair color and a variety of hair structures. These variables make it challenging for a robot to be consistently accurate; this can leave open the possibility for mistakes like damaging healthy hair grafts during the robotic hair transplant procedure.

At the time of this writing, the **ARTAS robotic hair transplant** technology still has one problem. It is not recommended for patients with curly hair; these patients often have to go with traditional FUT or FUE hair transplant surgery.

You may find some claims that the ARTAS robot will perform one hundred percent of the procedure without the help of a medical doctor or any medical personnel. This is not true; the ARTAS is only surgeon-assisted technology. This technology will most likely advance in the future. However, this chapter was designed

to give you some good things to be aware of
and questions to ask your doctor until it does.

Chapter Nine

Before and After

How to get the most out of your hair transplant procedure

Before your hair transplant, there are many things to keep in mind. First, the doctor is going to ask you about any vitamins or medications you are taking if you've had any illnesses, surgeries, or have any diagnosed illnesses.

They will also ask you to stop taking specific vitamins and supplements and to stop some habits like smoking and drinking alcohol several days before your procedure.

If you ever wanted to quit any bad habits like drinking alcohol or smoking, now would be a good time.

There's lots of advice out there about using pharmaceutical drugs that are on the market. Some of the most popular ones are Finasteride, Propecia, and Topical products like Rogaine that contain Minoxidil. I'm not a big fan of using any pharmaceutical drugs.

Just because the FDA approves a drug doesn't mean it's beneficial for you long-term. Many of these drugs are tested a few years in clinical trials before they are presented for sale and distribution to the USA market. The side effects on most warning labels should be an automatic red flag for any thinking person. I would rather focus on how to improve my health in a more natural way than relying on pharmaceutical drugs with nasty side effects. And I'm not talking any of that woo woo or hippie crap.

The fact is we live in one of the best times in history to take advantage of information coming from real scientists and doctors that care about you and I and less about making multi-million dollars in profits. Many of these professionals starting to break away from the dogma of junk science, hypotheses, studies, and research papers that have been pushed on us for years, many of which are often manipulated for big business industry profits.

Here are a few of the people I would highly recommend looking into. Their work is creating movements of people like you and me taking back control of our health.

Steven R Gundry, MD author of The Plant Paradox

Whim Hof is Dutch daredevil, the "Iceman" Known for the Whim Hof method

Naveen Jain, billionaire businessman is from India, the owner and founder of Voime for Gut Health

I'd like to share with you some of what I have not only learned, but have personally implemented, and as a result, have seen significant improvements in my health. Changes to help you absorb the proper nutrients for good health, but also in helping you avoid other chronic illnesses all of which contribute to the health of your hair.

I know this may sound a little cliché or even a bit arrogant. All I ask is that you hear me out with an open mind.

I believe health is like a puzzle. There are many pieces to this puzzle. However, each one of these puzzle pieces a bit of information. And just like a puzzle, sometimes we find a puzzle piece that we think is right and that fits. But as we keep looking, we see the exact puzzle piece that goes there. That is why we should keep an open mind; we may have to change that puzzle piece with the right one when we find it.

The information we get comes in many forms. What we must remember is this. There is not one doctor, scientist, medical professional, or friend that has all the exact correct information. They usually only have one or two pieces of the puzzle. Additionally, we are all made just a little bit different from one another.

I believe if we truly want to be healthy, it is our responsibility to put these puzzle pieces together. Doing this will enable us to put together our picture of health using the puzzle pieces that we see that fit for optimal health and wellness.

I want to cover some of the pieces of the puzzle that are universal to many of us.

Puzzle piece NO.1

Digestion

Most of us live in such a fast-paced environment where we find ourselves eating on the run, scarfing down our food quickly without even tasting it. I don't know about you, but I've never learned how to eat correctly to get the best digestion and absorption of all the nutrients I consume. I mean they don't teach it in school so it must not be a big deal... Right?

We have learned that our stomach has a bunch of acids in it to break down all of our food, so we can digest it. What if I told you digestion starts the second you smell food and put it in your mouth. That's right, research shows that the second we smell the food, we activate our salivary glands to produce more saliva and other chemical reactions inside our body that starts the preparation for receiving the food into our system. So we all do this naturally. However, the next part is the area in which most of us overlook, this is chewing our food correctly.

I heard a speech recently that had an interesting theory on the process of eating, and it makes a lot of sense. It went like this. "We should drink our food and chew our water." Let that sink in for a minute. It makes sense that we have teeth for a reason.

The goal of putting food into our mouth is to nourish our body. Have you ever heard the suggestion not to swallow certain pills such as vitamin B12? It is recommended that you put B12 under your tongue (sublingual) for proper absorption. The reason for this is that taking B12 Sublingual (under the tongue) is one of the quickest ways for it to get into our bloodstream.

Our mouth alone has hundreds, if not thousands, of different blood vessels. Our mouth is designed to not only break the food down with our teeth, but our saliva is also a big part of the digestion process. Our saliva alone contains special enzymes that help break down our food as we chew. The more we chew our food, the more saliva production we will have for proper digestion. If you make it a practice of chewing your food more before you swallow, it will be easier and more beneficial for your digestion.

If you're digesting your food correctly your body will absorb more nutrients not only from your mouth but through the rest of your digestive system as well. Chewing is one of the simplest things you can do that doesn't cost any money and can have a profound effect on your hair growth and your health because you are absorbing more of the nutrients you are consuming.

However, you don't want your body absorbing the wrong nutrients. Today the scientific information is almost unanimously concurring that our health starts in our gut.

That is why I highly recommend reading Dr. Steven Gundry's book -*The Plant Paradox*. After reading *The Plant Paradox* you will have a whole new understanding of how some so-called healthy foods can be the cause of lots of health issues.

Puzzle piece NO. 2

Stress and Anxiety

Stress can not only affect your hair growth or lack thereof but can also impact your health in many different ways.

This is one of the main reasons why you will often hear it recommended that you keep your stress levels low.

It is common in people that are extremely stressed actually to lose hair or even patches of hair. Stress starves the body of the necessary building blocks to maintain itself. So you may be thinking to yourself, how can stress cause that? Well, even though we live in a modern world, our bodies and brains are still very primitive.

Our primitive brain still deals with stress the way it did thousands of years ago. The way I like to think about it is to picture in your mind two different worlds. In one world, you live in a cave, and you have to go out to hunt for your food. The other world is a modern world where we have to go out and work for our food.

Let's take the first scenario - if you have to go out and hunt for your food. It's a little bit hard to picture in your mind what you would go through if you had to physically hunt for your food, especially if you were not using some modern device like a gun. So let's think about it this way - picture in your mind a large cat, let's say it's a cheetah. The cheetah sees another animal in the distance. The first thing that happens is, the brain focuses its eyes on the other animal. The large cat gets very still, it crouches down and starts to move slowly toward its prey. Getting ready to run, it gets closer to the ground, and then at the right moment, it takes off running as fast as it can. The large cat catches the animal, and now it has to kill it to have food. The struggle can go on for several minutes before the cat clutches it's jaws around its neck, draining the life of the other animal.

Now I want you to think about how intense just reading that was. Now, if we think about the animal, all of the energy in the animal's body went to its muscles. It's vision, it's breathing even changes making it 100% entirely focused on killing that animal. But when we think of this big cat, how long do you think it took the cheetah to kill the animal - maybe 10, 15, 20 minutes? Once the big cat made its kill, it still had some work to do; however, the hard part was done.

So when we think about it, the cheetah getting its food might not be much different than us. You see, we're made to handle short periods of stress just like the big cat.

The problem with most people today is, as we get into a state of constant stress without addressing it, our body goes into the same stressed condition the cat does when stalking its prey for food. Our breathing changes, our muscles tighten, and our body is tensed up. If we are in a constant environment of stress, it robs our body of the time it needs to rest and digest and remain healthy.

Being in this stressed state in combination with eating processed foods are depriving us of essential nutrients and having a profound effect on our body, causing a wide variety of health issues. Prolonged stress also leaves our body in a state where we find ourselves having a hard time regenerating because of lack of rest, and also leaves your whole body open to sickness and disease.

Puzzle piece NO 3
Food
The ancient Greek Physician Hippocrates was also known as the father of medicine; he is known for this famous quote, "let food be thy medicine and medicine be thy food."

Humanity has had significant achievements over the years. However, at the start of the industrial revolution, men like John D. Rockefeller pushed science into coming up with medicines that they could patent.

During this time, natural remedies were largely discredited. Don't get me wrong, some medicines save lives; however, many are overprescribed. What this has done to us as a society is that it has made us dependent on pharmaceutical drugs. It is many times the first place we look to find solutions to our health challenges.

The industrial revolution also brought in industrial style farms where just a few farms produced much of the food for the world. Doing so has drastically changed not only what food we eat, but the quality of the food as well.

Let's start with the food. Many of us grew up being taught to eat according to the food pyramid. All the grains and breads were at the bottom. Next, fruits and vegetables. Then meat and dairy and at the very top is fat, oils, and sweets.

To get an in-depth look at what foods can be harmful to you, many of which we have been taught are extremely beneficial, are actually hurting you. I would highly recommend reading
Dr. Stephen R Gundry's book
The Plant Paradox

With basic foods in the USA, you have many that are GMO also known as genetically modified organisms. And you also have non-GMO foods.

We still do not know the full effects of GMO food, in many countries around the world, there are laws either against producers of GMO food and many countries require food producers to disclose the GMO on the food label. But not here in the United States of America.

In many cases, GMO foods were created to withstand the harsh pesticides being sprayed on the vast majority of the crops in the USA. Most industrial crops use a pesticide that you may have heard of before called Round-Up. This product is made by Monsanto. Round-Up is a poisonous weed killer; however, many farmers use it for what they referred to as a desiccant for the crops. In other words, they're spraying Roundup on their crops in large amounts to dry them out faster so they can then be harvested at a quicker rate. This is a widely prevalent practice used by most industrial wheat farmers in the USA. I would encourage you to do your research on the effects of glyphosate on the human body.
At the time of this writing, there is a massive amount of lawsuits against the company Monsanto in the USA.

Not surprisingly, glyphosates are found in a large amount of the food what we eat. For this reason, it is highly recommended that you do your best to eat organic food. By law, organic food providers are certified and guarantee that their product is not contaminated with glyphosate or pesticides, therefore allowing you a better opportunity to gain the necessary benefits from the foods you eat.

Puzzle piece NO. 4
Food and Sleep
One of the biggest complaints I've heard is guys wondering why their results after their hair transplant are slower or not as good as others. One of the contributing factors to the quality of your results will largely depend on your body's ability to heal itself. Our bodies are continually regenerating themselves 24 hours a day. Here are a few things you can do to assist your body in its regenerative healing process. Remember, it's the small things done over and over that make a big difference.

First, let's look at your sleep. Getting quality sleep is vital when it comes to allowing the body to heal properly, especially after a hair transplant procedure. However, this is easier said than done. Here are some helpful tips:

I recommended not to eat anything 3 to 4 hours before you go to bed. Why? Your body will have 3 to 4 hours before you go to sleep to start digesting your food. As we discussed earlier, your blood has specific properties that heal the body. However, if we eat just before we sleep, our body will concentrate blood around the stomach to aid in digestion and is forced to take time away from healing itself while you are sleeping, therefore delaying the ability for the body to heal.

Puzzle piece NO. 5
Effects of Smoking and Alcohol

When you go in for a hair transplant, the doctor will recommend that you stop smoking and drinking alcohol several days before your procedure. One of the main reasons for this is that the body has a harder time healing if you are a smoker or have alcohol in your system.

Smoking disrupts the oxygen available to heal your body's cells and does not allow the cells to function correctly. Smoking can decrease the amount of oxygen in our blood and affect circulation. Anything that affects the blood circulation to the scalp can reduce the rate of healing and cause the hair follicles that are transplanted to suffer or even die. Remember that the hair follicles will be removed and have to live outside of the body for a short period before transplanting is complete. Smoking before and after a hair transplant can make the hair follicles weak, which could lead to a reduction of successfully transplanted hair follicles. Smoking can also increase bleeding during the surgery because of the nicotine in the body. So if you've ever wanted to stop smoking, now would be a good time to quit altogether. If not, at least follow the before and after instructions from the doctor.

Alcohol is another substance that disturbs the body and its ability to heal correctly. Alcohol turns into sugar in your bloodstream. It's known to cause inflammation, and that causes your blood veins to dilate. When combined with dehydration, it can result in alcohol-related swelling. Excessive swelling can compromise the effectiveness of your hair transplant and reduce healing, delaying the growth of new hair.

Alcohol also increases bleeding; it makes the blood thinner putting you at a higher risk of excessive bleeding during and after the surgery. Excessive bleeding can make recovery time much longer. In some instances, doctors will have to stop the transplant surgery and re-schedule for the next day.

So be sure to follow your doctor's advice, when it comes to drinking alcohol. Because if not, you might become THAT GUY, that finds yourself complaining about why your results aren't as good as everyone else.

Puzzle piece NO. 6
Vitamins & Minerals & Supplements
Here are some recommended Vitamins and Supplements to aid in your hair transplant success:

Saw Palmetto: For hair loss and thinning, Saw Palmetto is useful to block DHT hormone or dihydrotestosterone. Various types of Saul Palmetto supplements are being combined with other vitamins and minerals and are being specifically labeled as a DHT hormone blocker. I'm a firm believer in taking vitamins and minerals that are combined into one pill. In the right combination, they can be more effective than taking a stand-alone supplement.

Pygeum: For hair loss and thinning. Pygeum is said to be better than Saw Palmetto for blocking the DHT hormones. Some say it's as effective as the pharmaceutical drug finasteride.

Biotin: Helps thicken the hair. Biotin is an essential B vitamin. Stand-alone vitamins are not always absorbed well. I like Biotin supplements that are mixed with other essential vitamins and minerals. My personal favorite is a Biotin supplement called "Extra Strength Hair Skin and Nails" made by Natures Bounty. You can find it at Costco for a great price.

Magnesium: Helps thicken and strengthen the hair. Magnesium is essential for protein synthesis and over 300 functions inside the human body. Magnesium is another mineral that is more effective when combined with other vitamins and minerals. My personal favorite is called "Natural Calm Plus Calcium" made by Natural Vitality. It can be purchased on Amazon for a great price.

Collagen: Collagen helps thicken and strengthen hair. Collagen is made up of essential amino acids. It can be found in a powder supplement or bone broth in liquid or powder form.

Aloe Vera Juice: Aloe Vera Juice helps naturally strengthen and thicken your hair. It contains polysaccharides and can be found in juice or gel form. It is recommended to drink one cup of Aloe Vera Juice per day.

Rosemary Oil: Rosemary Oil helps with hair thinning and hair loss. It has been known to slow down or even stop DHT hormones, dihydrotestosterone when applied directly to the scalp. Some recommend mixing it with olive oil, then applying it to the scalp.

Omega 3 Fatty Acids: Omega 3 Fatty Acids strengthen your hair and the recommended dose is 1000mg- 3000mg per day. Omega 3 Fatty Acids can be found in pills or liquid form. Flaxseed oil, cod liver oil or fish oil are all forms of Omega 3 Fatty Acids. It is also found in salmon and other fish. Anytime you purchase fish it's important to look for wild-caught, not farm-raise. Remember "you are what you eat" so if a fish has been farmed and fed corn and other harmful foods, that is what you will be eating instead of the fish's natural diet from the sea or ocean.

IN SUMMARY

I want to approach this the way physicists approach problems. They start by breaking down all of the basic principles. Once these basic principles are broken down, you can decide in which order to put things back together. Most often, this will solve almost any problem in a simplistic and easy to understand way.

So in this particular instance, the problem we are attempting to solve is hair loss, hair thinning, and male pattern baldness.
I think we could all agree that we are all after one result - that is to have thicker, healthier natural-looking hair... And, of course, more of it!!!

Next, we will focus on hair transplant procedures - beginning with traveling to the appointments.
When it comes to the health of your hair, there are many factors we will look at.

Chapter Ten

Travel Tips

AIRLINE TICKETS:

Sky Scanner is a great website to get discounted international airline tickets, access the link to their website at www.TheHairTransplantBook.com/Support-Links You can also set up an alert so that if there are any changes to the price of tickets for the dates you are considering, it will alert you via email. It's wise to use an incognito window if you visit the site multiple times so that the website cannot track your visits.

Many times when travel websites see you have visited the site multiple times, they will manipulate the price to be higher, costing you more money. If you are not familiar with incognito windows or tabs, I would recommend doing a search on YouTube for instructions on how to open an incognito window; it will be worth the education. Once you learn this, it will be a simple but effective tool to use.

REFUNDABLE OR NON REFUNDABLE TICKETS:

When purchasing airline tickets, I would recommend using a credit card, not a debit card. The reason for this is that many credit cards have travel insurance built into your benefits as a cardholder. Before using your credit card, you can call the 800 number on the back of the card and ask if they provide any Travel Insurance. If not, you can get supplemental insurance from companies like AIG. However, be careful about purchasing extra insurance through travel websites, when buying your airline tickets. Many of the travel website insurance companies have various loopholes to get around when requesting that they pay out on claims. When taking an international flight, it is recommended that you check-in 24 hours before your trip to be sure there are no changes to your itinerary. You can check-in from their website or phone app. Many times this is the best time to ask for an upgrade. It is also best to get to the airport early to give yourself plenty of time to get through security and to the gate. Some non-refundable tickets can have hefty fees associated with missing any legs of your flight.

DISCOUNTED PARKING:

Almost every airport will have short and long-term parking areas.

The following is a travel hack - we use to get discounted and sometimes free parking using this travel hack. Depending on the airport we travel from, we will contact the different hotels around the airport, many of these hotels will let you park there for FREE if you stay in the hotel the night before your departure. There are even some hotels that have special designated parking areas for travelers that charge a fraction of the price the airport charges, as low as USD 5.00 per day. You park your car at their hotel and take their shuttle to the airport for FREE.

PASSPORT:

Always have a picture copy or printed copy of your passport as a backup just in case with you and one at home with your emergency contact. When you get your passport, pay a little extra for the Passport ID card. Then when traveling around during the day you will be able to leave your Passports locked in the safe in your room, and if necessary can still prove your identity with the Passport ID. In many cases, only one person in your party needs to carry it, and it looks similar to a driver's license in the USA.

TRAVEL LIGHT:

In our family, we have become accustomed to traveling light. Each of us carries a backpack and a small carry-on suitcase. Traveling light helps your long-anticipated adventure from becoming a travel nightmare. Our saying is, "checked bags are lost bags." This is especially true if you are taking multiple flights to reach your final destination. If you're having a hard time making it to your connecting flight, there's a good chance your luggage will too. So many experts on traveling abroad and even in the USA suggest packing light as a way to really enjoy your trip, but not having too many bags or things to keep track of while you are away from home.

TRAVEL VISA:

Not all countries require a travel Visa.

If you're from the USA, you can look at the State Department website to determine whether you will need a Travel Visa for the country you're traveling to. Some require that you apply for travel documents at the Embassy or Consulate. In our example, we are going to Istanbul, Turkey, and Turkey does require a travel Visa. However, it is effortless to get it online, and it costs right at USD 20.00. You can go to the following website to get your e-Visa for Turkey.

www.TheHairTransplantBook.com/Support-Links

PACKING:

Be sure when packing you check the weather forecast and the local clothing customs for the communities you will be visiting. Things can be very different in other parts of the world, and you want to be considerate and have safe travels when abroad. DON'T OVERPACK! Bring clothes that mix and match and double-check the airline luggage requirements. The airlines will also have weight requirements for your bags that you should be aware of. Have all of your important travel documents with you and close at all times. You may want to skip the lace-up shoes and belts for your days at the airport. This will help you get through security faster if you wear shoes that come on and off easily and also no belt. Otherwise, you will probably have to take them off to get through the security checkpoint. Remember to download the WhatApp App for international texting and phone calls, and download any Google Maps you need before you get there in case there is not a strong internet connection.

CURRENCY/ MONEY EXCHANGE:

Never carry a lot of cash.

Let your credit card companies and your bank know you'll be traveling abroad. Doing a simple search for travel wallets on Amazon, you'll find many options for concealing your cash and belongings under your clothes for safety while in a foreign country. You are keeping your cash safe from the common scam in most countries of being pickpocketed.

CREDIT CARDS ABROAD:

You will need to call your credit card companies before you leave the country to let them know the dates and countries you will be visiting. Also, check on foreign transaction fees that could be incurred by using your credit card abroad. If you plan to use your credit card for any part of your hair transplant procedure you will need to see what extra fee the clinic charges for the use of a credit card. You will also have to confirm which credit cards they will accept for payment, as not all are accepted.

CELL PHONE SERVICE ABROAD:

When traveling abroad, it is essential to check with your cellular phone provider to check on your service, calls and texting options, wifi options, and any additional charge you will experience while you are away. We were pleasantly surprised that while we are in Turkey, we will have cell service, free texting, and call(s) will cost USD 0.25 per minute through our T-Mobile Cellular Phone Plan.

TRANSPORTATION:

If you decide to go to Turkey for your hair transplant, all the clinics we spoke to will provide transportation to and from the airport and between each visit to the clinic for your appointments included in your price. If you do have to take a taxi when exploring the city, it is best to confirm with your hotel how much you should have to pay for each destination. One of the known scams in Turkey is the taxi drivers spotting tourists and charging exorbitant amounts for taxi fares. Then it is recommended to take exact change for your taxi ride, or at least do not pay your taxi fare with large money bills.

BEST TIMES TO VISIT:

You want to confirm with your clinic of choice if the dates you are planning to come are available. I would recommend not to have a hair transplant procedure done during their local holidays. Also the clinic we will be using sent us a confirmation letter with our appointment date and time so that we will have all that in writing before we ever leave home.

SAFETY:

If you are from the USA you can check the US State Department's website. At the time of this writing, Turkey is a LEVEL 3. If the US State Department issues any travel bans, many times, it is easier to get a refund on your airfare. If you do decide to travel to Turkey for your hair transplant, remember that Turkey is a NATO Ally. You can find the link to enroll in the Smart Traveler Enrollment Program at our support page:

<u>www.TheHairTransplantBook.com/Support-Links</u>   It will log your travel days and location for the US Government so that if you need assistance while you are away, you will be able to access help quicker. Despite the best planning, things can go wrong, and they offer 24-hour, 7-day week support if needed.

Chapter Eleven

Financing Your Hair Transplant Procedure

So now, with the realization of how affordable a hair transplant can be, you may be thinking, OKAY, I'm ready to pull the trigger, but I need funds. Well, there is the option of financing your procedure, just like I did with my first hair transplant. Since you're looking at funding less than USD 5000 for the hair transplant, there are several options out there.

Before we start looking for a credit card or loan, I would highly recommend reviewing your credit score. Most of the time, there are small things you can do to improve your credit score before you apply for any credit.

Let's answer the following questions first:
1.   What's the easiest way to get your credit score raised?

2.   Will it cost me any money to work on my credit?

3.   Do I have to pay someone to work on my credit for me?

No, No, and No!!!

First, you will need to create a Credit Karma Account, you can find the link at our support page:
www.thehairtransplantbook.com/Support-Links
This costs zero to set up. Credit Karma gives you the ability to monitor two of the three major credit monitoring bureaus, TransUnion and Equifax. They also have resources on their website to review and dispute any inaccurate information being reported on your credit report. If you dispute items and get them removed, it will bring up your credit score. Even simple things like the incorrect spelling of your name, address, or other basic information, dates on accounts, or inaccurate amounts. The best part of Credit Karma is that they will recommend and pre-approve you for credit cards that you have a good chance of receiving. This is very helpful, so you're not wasting your time getting unnecessary dings

against your Credit when applying for a bunch of cards that may or may not deny you.

Next, this step involves finding somebody that you trust -This could be a relative, a direct family member, or even a close friend. Here's how it works: you need to find a person with a credit card that they have had for at least a few years - the longer, the better. They need to be trustworthy because their payment history on this account should show that it is paid regularly, and also they need to plan on paying it regularly moving forward. The next step is to see if they are willing to have you added to that specific credit card account. Once you get approved to be added to the credit card account, the credit card company will send a card with your name on it. Now they don't have to give you a card; they can keep it or toss it. But what happens is a portion of -if not all of the credit limit and history will then be reported to the credit bureaus as part of your history, giving you years of good payment history.

Doing this will automatically raise your credit utilization and or available credit and will also show years of good payment history. Even though you may not have access to that card, your name and social security number have been attached to the account, and you gain all the history of that account. I have used this tip personally with my two daughters, and they have both been able to enter their young adulthood with credit scores in the high 700+ Credit Score based on our payment history for the account they were added to.

You might have to wait a month or so to see changes. However, once you've set up your Credit Karma account, you can check your score every day if you want. Once your credit score has gone up, there's a good chance you can apply for and get a credit card that will cover your entire trip and procedure. If you want more than just a few thousand in credit, you can apply for several cards at once. By doing it this way, the other cards will not see that you've applied for multiple cards because they were submitted simultaneously of each other. I would also be looking to see if there are any 0% interest introductory rate credit cards. Many cards will give you a 0% interest for 12 to 18 months, which would allow you to have the procedure interest free for the first year and pay it off quicker.

If you have a good to excellent credit somewhere in the 650 to 750 range, I suggest applying for one my favorite cards, the Chase Sapphire Reserve card.

www.TheHairTransplantBook.com/Support-Links

This card has an annual fee associated with it, however, the moment you booked any travel on this card Chase will immediately credit back to your account the majority of the annual fee. This card also has some really great perks like travel insurance, up to three points on travel and dining, a welcome bonus offer of 60,000 points or more, reimbursement on TSA pre-check, and a private travel booking website. However, one of the best things my wife and I like about the Chase Sapphire Reserve Card is they give you an additional membership card at no cost too.

Priority Pass Select Members have access to over 1,300 airport lounges around the world, including hundreds across North and South America. This exclusive membership alone is a USD 500 value. Your membership will get you and a guest in free of charge. Many of these Priority lounges have free food, free alcohol, and nonalcoholic beverages along with free Wi-Fi, showers, and many other perks. A quiet lounge to relax between flights.

Chapter Twelve

The Best Decision

I want you to make the best-informed decision when it comes to your hair transplant.
We have created a Secret Private Facebook group:
Here is your invitation to connect here
Access our private community:
www.TheHairTransplantBook.com/Support-Links

This will be a safe community to ask questions, share experiences and see me walk through my entire hair transplant experience via video in Istanbul, Turkey November 2019.

This will be a private community that will allow us to have real conversations, share results, and discuss how to get and maintain the best hair transplant results in the world.

We will be able to help you do your due diligence when deciding all the details for your hair transplant journey so that you will have a smooth, successful experience.

We will be negotiating discounts for members of our community so that you will be getting the best deals not only close to home, but also on your journey abroad if that is what you choose for your hair transplant procedure.

We are building and will supply alliance partners close to home for each of our members for PRP treatments, Micro Pigmentation, and hair clinics so that you will have all the information in front of you to make the best decisions moving forward in your hair restoration journey.

You will see tons of Social Proof and will be encouraged to connect with fellow members of our private community to assist you with questions and challenges.

Chapter Thirteen

How I made my final decision

When I started my research, my goal was to get the best hair transplant possible. I wanted someone good. I didn't want to feel just okay about it; I wanted the best experience and the best results! Thirteen years ago, I felt the experience was okay, not excellent. My first hair transplant procedure was only a thousand hair grafts. This time I am equipped with knowledge that will make all the difference in my results. Now that I'm over 43, I want it to take years off my physical appearance with my next hair transplant!

So when I first started researching to find the best hair transplant clinic, the first thing that came to mind was, "damn - this is going to cost at least USD 25,000.00 to USD 30,000.00 to get my hair done the way I want it. Then my business mind kicked in, and I asked myself the questions - how can I get the best quality, the best results, and the best price for my next hair transplant? Suddenly, I remembered years ago we worked with a gentleman that had a medical tourism company in Kuala Lumpur, Malaysia. So in my mind, I knew what was possible. I recommended to my wife Rachel that we start looking into the possibility of finding a company outside of the USA for my hair transplant procedure.

As we started our search, there was one country in particular that kept showing up. We were beginning to see a pattern of not only the specific country, but all the arrows were pointing to a particular city - that city was none other than Istanbul, Turkey.

That's right, Istanbul, Turkey. Istanbul is the largest city in Turkey, boasting a population of over 15 million people. The country of Turkey alone has nearly 350 hair transplant clinics, the majority of which are in Istanbul. Just a few years ago, in 2016, it was reported that more than 60,000 medical travelers from around the world that visit Turkey are for hair loss treatments.

What about the quality?
Turkey is known for its expert doctors, not only for hair transplants but plastic surgery and other cosmetic procedures.

Through our research, we found that many Turkish doctors specialize in the latest treatments and technology, and have spent many years honing their skills. We also noticed that many of these doctors are teaching at international conferences, and speaking on the latest techniques that are shaping the hair transplant industry.

It even appears that the government of Turkey has recognized the importance of sustaining the growth of this lucrative industry. Their reputation is excellent, and the level of quality is at the highest standard. The Turkish Ministry of Health audits all hospitals twice a year to ensure they meet the quality, safety, and service that they've set forth in their local laws.

Many hospitals in Istanbul, Turkey also have high International Accreditations, like JCI – Joint Commission International, which ensures that hospitals are up to international standards. Turkey has the third-highest number of JCI accredited hospitals in the world. Some of the best hair transplant clinics work directly out of these hospitals.

It is essential to choose the right clinic to avoid a bad experience. Here are a few things to look for when doing your due diligence.

First, ask for proof that the doctor is licensed. In many clinics, the technicians will be doing a large percentage of the hair transplant procedure. This is not a bad thing; I would recommend asking how much experience the medical technician has that will be performing most of your hair transplant procedure - the longer, the better. With the clinic we chose, the technicians have 7 to 8 years of experience doing hair transplants. Just remember, from my example of having an overpriced hair transplant in the USA, the actual medical technicians extracted each of the hair follicles from the strip the doctor removed. The technicians also implanted each hair follicle after the doctor opened the small channels in the recipient area at the top of my head. I forgot to mention this before, so I'll say it now, the medical technicians extracted all the hair follicles from the strip taken from my head, after that the doctor made the small cuts in my scalp referred to as channels. The doctor began swiftly stabbing my head with some small surgical tool; I remember the doctor counting each hair channel he opened. He was counting so fast that you could barely hear him say the actual numbers. He almost sounded like an auctioneer taking bids from around the room, blabbering numbers I could scarcely understand. Remembering, I can hardly imagine that he opened each channel as methodically and meticulously as possible. The whole time I was thinking, I can't believe I'm paying USD 9000.00 for this. Can you imagine?

Chapter Fourteen

Process of Elimination

With hundreds of clinics to choose from, it was time to get to work.

There are lots of medical travel coordination companies that will help you with your medical travel package. We spent weeks going through dozens of websites, narrowing down what we consider the best companies. Taking notes, reading reviews, reading company websites, looking up before and after pictures, and identifying congruences and incongruencies.

Several weeks later, we were able to narrow our search down to 15 hair transplant clinics. Next, we started to send text and picture messages to each hair transplant clinic through WhatsApp. WhatsApp is an international texting App owned by Facebook that is a great way to communicate with people all over the world for no cost. This app also allows you to make international phone calls for free. Once we connected, the clinics requested photos and necessary medical information so they could provide recommendations and a somewhat solid estimate of what we would expect to pay for the hair transplant.

Here is an example of a quote we got back, including the pictures we sent them to receive pricing. They require pictures of each angle of your head, including each side, front, back and top to give the most complete quote. If the donor area does not look strong, they may request pictures of your beard and chest area so see the other options for hair transplantation.

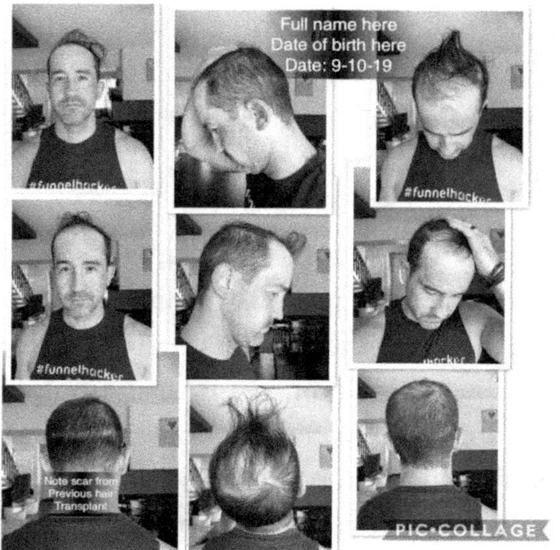

Diagnosis of your case by Dr. E is :

- Technique: Micro FUE

- Minimum number of Follicles expected to be extracted: 3000-4000 grafts and this number might increase to a higher number depending on the density of donor area

- Coverage ratio: 100 % of the baldness area, we will redraw the front hairline and give you the highest density possible in all the transplanted areas

- Hair Supplement: we will apply PRP injection + Mesotherapy injection during your operation to nourish your hair follicles

 - Guaranty: you will receive a guaranty letter stating the follicles will not lose hair once they have united with the skin

The procedure plan is :

First   Arrival Day: you will have the consultation with The doctor and the blood test

Second Day: will be the operation day

Third day: for taking rest after the operation ...

Fourth day: for bandage removal and hair washing

(Before and After Pictures Sent)

(Doctors Credentials sent)

The Package price is: USD 2900

The discounted price of the package: USD 2300.00

Package will include:

- Your hair transplant operation is done under Dr. E supervision*. who is a certified doctor by the ministry of health in Turkey and a member of ISHRS (International Society of Hair Restoration Surgery)

- Your Transportation in Istanbul between the Airport to the hospital and the hotel.

- Your hotel reservation for 3 nights in a 5-star hotel that is located in a touristic area
- PRP session and Mesotherapy for follicles strengthening and hair densifying.
- Guaranty Certificate that your operation will be successful and you will have a healthy normal look.
- A Medical bag that includes a shampoo and lotion and after operation medication
Not included to the package:
- extended stay in the hotel
- flight ticket
Instructions before the operation :
- Patient must stop using pain killer, aspirins, alcohol, green tea, and drugs 5 days before the procedure
- Smokers must not smoke more than 5 cigarettes for 2 days at least before the operation day
We only need a screenshot of the flight ticket to confirm your booking, So If you want to book the flight, please let me know the dates of the arrival and departure and then I will check the hospital schedule and give you the confirmation.

Chapter Fifteen

Bonus

Below is the list of questions that we used to qualify each potential hair transplant clinic.

1.   Do they meet our standards for using all the current, best up-to-date hair transplant technology?

Primarily, we are looking for companies that offered DHI (Direct Hair Implant) as their standalone method for hair transplants. Or a combination of DHI in conjunction with the traditional hair implantation method using a sapphire tool to create the hair channels. As for hair extraction, my preference is Micro FUE, and no use of the artist robotic or Neo graft Extraction for my next hair transplant.

2.   Next, does the doctor have ISHRS "International Society of Hair Restoration Surgery," training and certifications?

3.   Is the hair procedure performed in an actual hospital?

In Istanbul, the government tightly regulates their medical tourism. Turkish laws require cosmetic surgeries to be performed inside a licensed hospital; the hospitals are equipped to deal with emergencies that could arise during a medical operation.

4.   Is the hospital a JCI-USA accredited hospital?

5.   Do they charge extra for a second day?

Many clinics will charge an additional fee for a second day to get more hair grafts transplanted. This may be necessary if you require a more significant number of hair grafts. I have seen some cases of people getting 6000 to 7000 grafts. Most of the clinics are comfortable doing 4000 to 5000 hair grafts per day. If your donor area is weak, they may recommend taking it from the lower neck or beard area, the chest, or even from your back. The hair transplant clinic I chose has a base price of USD 2100.00; however, if you require a second day, it would be an additional USD 600.00.

6.   Do they offer PRP (Platelet Rich Plasma) with the hair transplant procedure?

It is essential because with PRP treatment, the results of the newly transplanted hair will significantly improve.

7.   Do they offer or include in their quote needle-free numbing /anesthesia?

Some companies will charge an extra USD 200.00 to USD 300.00 just for this benefit.

8.   Do they offer an aftercare hair transplant package included their quote, and what do they include in it?

It is essential to know the contents of any aftercare package that is offered. Some will include the aftercare package in the quote, and some will offer it to you only after the procedure for an additional cost. I've seen these aftercare packages range anywhere from USD 150.00 to USD 500.00.

9. Do they have an excellent online presence and reputation?

Be aware of any negative feedback regarding the clinic or doctor via videos, blog forums, or any other verified references. We looked at and used Google searches, Google business search, social media groups, and anything found posted on any of the medical network sites.

10. Do they have a high review rating?

Once again, we compared reviews from Google searches, Google maps business search, company website, social media, and any other reviews found posted on multiple medical network sites.

11 Are reviews reliable, and do they look legitimate?

Google makes this especially easy. The reviews usually have the person's profile attached. By glancing at their profile, you can quickly see how many other reviews they wrote. If they have some excellent reviews and some bad reviews of their various experiences with other businesses, this is usually a good indication their reviews are legitimate.

12. Are there any legitimate patient complaints?

One thing I like to do is look at all of the negative reviews first. Many times there will be people complaining about ridiculous things that have nothing to do with the quality or level of service they received from the clinic.

13. How many procedures do they perform per month on average?

I asked this question only after narrowing down to our two favorite clinics. I did not want to have a clinic that was pumping out hundreds of people a week like an assembly line. The clinic we finally chose performed 2 to 3 procedures per day.

14.   Do they have a guarantee?

The company we chose has a guarantee consisting of redoing the hair transplant procedure at no cost if the transplanted hair fails. You would have to pay for another flight and hotel, but everything else would at no charge if the hair transplant procedure had to be redone. However, you would not want to use a guarantee like this unless absolutely necessary, because you only have a certain amount of donor area, and once it's gone, it's gone! A hair transplant is not like getting a routine haircut.

15.   Do they have a translator available to you day and night?

This is important because many do not speak fluent English. Many clinics will assign you a translator that will help you from the initial quote through the completion of the hair transplant procedure.

16.   Are they putting us up in a five-star hotel without us having to request it?

This was important to me just for the simple fact that most of the time, quality likes quality. Additionally, you will be spending more time in your hotel room during your rest and recovery time after your procedure. Side note, I was going to pay our hotel with credit card points; however, the cost I would've paid was USD 60.00 more per night than the price that the clinic was able to get us, so I just had them keep the hotel in the package for my hair transplant.

17.   Is transportation included?

Every clinic should be providing transportation as a standard option. This transportation should be as follows: transportation from the airport when you arri.ve at your hotel, then from your hotel back and forth to the clinic throughout your stay. And lastly, from your hotel to the airport when you depart.

18.   Will they allow you to pay with a credit card?

Most clinics will allow you to pay with a credit card. The clinic I chose added a charge of an extra 8% up and above their quoted price for my hair transplant. So with a credit card, it will cost an additional USD168.00. I could carry around the cash amount with me, but I figure the USD168.00 is like having extra insurance. Oh yeah, and they also said they don't accept American Express only Visa and MasterCard, so this will be an additional detail to verify when you are choosing a clinic, and you plan to use a specific payment type.

19.   How does the price compare to other clinics for the same number of hair grafts?

For the most part, the clinics we contacted quoted prices anywhere from USD1500.00 to USD 2500.00. Also, the cost varies if you need a mega session; this usually consists of a second day. For a second day, we were getting back quotes for anywhere from USD 200.00 to USD 600.00, still, some charged more for having the doctor create the hair channels and/or place the hair follicles via DHI in the recipient area of the head. With some clinics, it could cost you as much as an additional USD 500.00 to USD1000.00 if you request this specifically for the doctor to perform the hair transplant procedure.

The clinic we finally chose passed for all the above questions.

Chapter Sixteen

Final thoughts

In conclusion, I would like to thank you for taking the time to read this book. Whatever road you decide to take along your journey to getting back your hair, I hope that this book has assisted you in getting the best results that are perfect for you.

As I'm writing the end of this book, I am only a few days away from catching my flight to Istanbul, Turkey. We booked round-trip tickets through the Skyscanner.com. From Colorado Springs, Colorado to Istanbul, Turkey, the airline flights we found had two stops, and each way is right at 20 hours of travel time. Going, we fly from Colorado Springs, Colorado USA to Chicago, Illinois USA to Amsterdam and then to Istanbul. Our return flight from Istanbul to Paris, France to Chicago, Illinois USA to Colorado Springs Colorado, USA.

The cost of each round trip airline ticket was USD 680.00.

Since we've been doing a lot of flying lately, this time, we decided to purchase our TSA Pre-Check Membership, you can find the link to join at our support page
www.TheHairTransplantBook.com/Support-Links
The TSA Pre-check membership allows you to get through airport security quicker without having to take your shoes off or remove your computer or liquids from your carry on bags. TSA's precheck membership cost is USD 85.00 each and lasts five years. A bonus is our Chase Sapphire Reserve credit card covers the TSA membership with a Credit back of USD100.00 toward the cost of this membership. I mentioned this card before in the finance section of this book. Here is a link if you would like to check that Chase Sapphire Reserve Card out and look at all the added benefits. You gotta love that!
www.TheHairTransplantBook.com/Support-Links

I chose a clinic that is recommending I get 3500 hair grafts transplanted. They agreed to do what they call a hybrid treatment for my hair transplant. The hair extraction method used for my procedure will be micro FUE. The hair implantation method used will be a combination of DHI and Sapphire blade. They are also going to administer PRP and Mesotherapy with B-complex (Vitamin B1, B2, B6, B12) with the hair transplant procedure. The medical package for my hair transplant also includes a three-night stay at The Elysium Istanbul, Turkey, a five-star hotel with full breakfast each day we are there. My package also includes all transportation to and from the airport and from the hotel to the hospital each day.

The Clinic will perform a blood test before the procedure to ensure there are no issues they need to know about that could disrupt the hair transplant procedure or affect my results in any way.
They are also providing a medical care package that includes a special head pillow, antibiotics, pain relievers, shampoo, and lotion.

As you can imagine, I'm very excited and can hardly wait to have all my hair back. This is going to be a massive deal for me. I can tell from looking through all of the clinics before and after pictures that my results should be ten times better than I had with the first hair transplant that cost me over USD 9000.00 with no extra perks like hotel, food, or transportation.

With that said, this is the reason I'm writing this book. Simply because when I first discovered how a life-changing procedure is within arms reach to the average income person, I had to share. I believe a hair transplant like this can be genuinely life-changing because it has the ability to put that sparkle back in your eye, that smile back on your face, and it can give you back the confidence you may have lost. I genuinely believe at the end of the day all of the benefits you gain will make you a healthier person as well.

We look forward to welcoming you into our Private Community to support and inspire you on your personal journey. Visit the link below for access:
www.TheHairTransplantBook.com/Support-Links

THE STORY CONTINUES…
Get Instant Access to
"The Procedure ISTABUL"
The Sequel to The Hair Transplant
www.TheHairTransplantBook.com/Support-Links

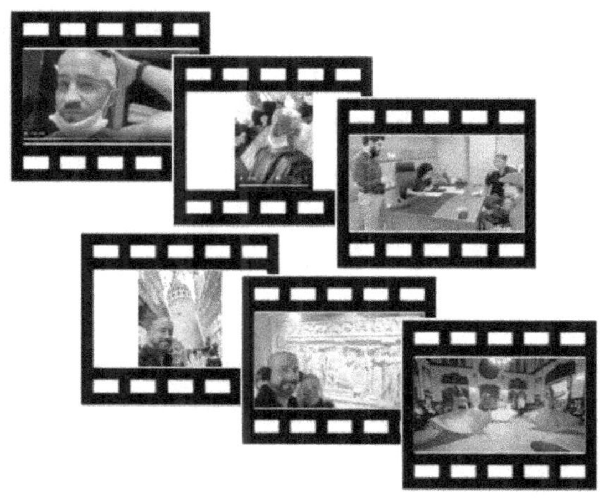

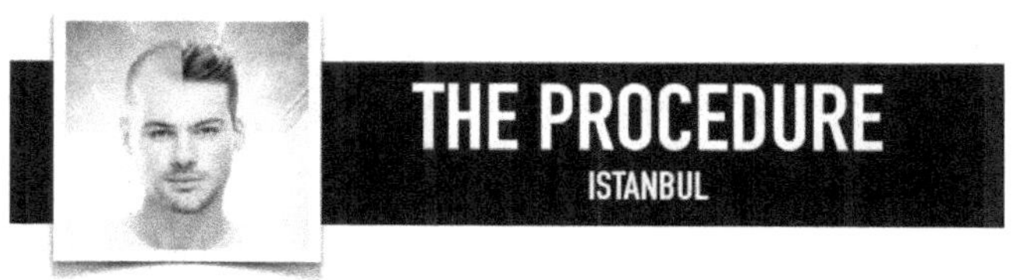
THE PROCEDURE
ISTANBUL

Author's bio:

Jamison Haponenko, a busy serial entrepreneur had his first hair transplant 13 years ago. At that time most of his time was focused on growing a thriving glass company he started. Being extremely busy he neglected to do all the research necessary when it came to discovering all the options available to him. Thinking that bigger might be better he decided to go with a large, highly recognized company to do his fist procedure. And the results were, let's just say okay... So 2 years ago he decided he was ready for a second hair transplant. However, this time he was on a mission. Over the last two years, he has spent countless hours in research and has consulted with industry leaders from around the world. All in an effort to find the best hair transplant results possible. This book will take you along his journey as he travels from blindly following the crowd to taking control and finding the best quality results at a mind-blowingly low price.

NOTES: